ESSAYS ON PERSONALITY

I0483882

Dr. Antonio Ridaura Aldana

To
Geraldine
Who is my reason for living

Homeopathy has always been the target of many different reactions. It is an undeniable fact that it has developed as an answer to many diseases and ailments of the human being. it is a science that is constantly evolving and being studied, it also intends to accurately respond to the essence of human beings.

Being aware of this diversity and giving a precise and reliable meaning to the human being, Dr. Antonio Ridaura classified the 8 personalities which are the result of a genome and are crucial to achieve healing.

Dr, Antonio Ridaura graduated from the Free School of Homeopathy in 1980. He was a pathology and histology assistant of this institution which golden era was built by masters like Dr. Landeta Siguenza, Dr. Jesus Diaz Barriga, Dr. Alejandro Rodriguez Mejia, Martin Vergara Sosa among others who do not come to mind in this moment. Because of them (mentors of doctors of homeopathy), Dr. Ridaura was a general practitioner of the Higinio G. Perez Hospital. He was a professor in CONALEP Ejido Puebla in 1983 and taught "human relations and science methodology". He was also an undergraduate scholarship holder of the Health Center in Mexicali, Baja California.

Alternating all kinds of services for a year and a half, Ridaura lectured on high risk pregnancy, shock and bleeding topics to dentistry interns and nurses. Nowadays, he has been working as a private doctor for 30 years and owns a homeopathic medicine foundation, of which he is the main founding member.

Essays on Personality
Dr. Antonio Ridaura Aldana

Life and are oriented insofar as their own variables that are developed psychologically.

And here is when the doctor plays his role, guiding this personality and determining which the controlling substance is: this was the starting point of Essays on Personality. Thus, the descriptive listing made by Dr. Antonio Ridaura about the great variety of medicine that establishes his therapeutic approach, i which is condensed in this book, as a result of years of experience and through a particular research method, reminds us of the founder of homeopathic medicine, Dr. Samuel Hahnemann.

Mario Ridaura
BA in Philosophy

During his shift through the general medicine hall at Higinio G. Pérez Hospital, whenever Dr. Jaramillo looked into his briefcase to give one of his patients any kind of medication and someone asked him "what did you just give him/her?" he answered "study buddy".

Those were the moments when one felt relief in the presence of the clinic moment of Dr. Jaramillo who was in full command of all knowledge. And that phrase "study buddy' chased me for over 20 years.

Today, I have finally started with that "study buddy' and this essay has been created.

How can I forget the words of Dr. Rodriguez Mejia? There were around 117 students in his class and he always stated: "I would be satisfied if just 5 of you graduated and became homeopathic physicians". I think he was not mistaken; his example planted in all of us the desire just like Martin Vergara and others, to become part of the golden era of our school.

Antonio Ridaura

CONTENTS

1 Natrum Muriaticum 1

2 Phosphorous..7

3 Sepia Oficinalis 11

4 Silicea Terra 15

5 Nux Vomica 23

6 Pulsatilla Nigricans 29

7 Arsenicum Album 39

8 Lycopodium Clavatum....................................43

Appendix I 53

Apendix II 57

Introduction

Why prescribe according to the personality of the patient?
Personality always reigns over the biotype. Homeopathy Darwin.

The ancient Greek knowledge of medication was
obtained while traveling to Babylon, Egypt, India and Crete.
The origins of medicine are related to a legend about a
connection between religions and healing. The priests
(called Aesculapius priests, the Greek God of medicine)
controlled the healing ceremonies performed in temples
built in his honor. Eventually, the term Aesculapius priests
developed a new meaning, doctor. V

Miasma (from the Greek miasma: dirt, dust, infect)
means gas or foul mist which comes from waterholes or
decomposed matter; emanation coming from sick bodies,
lurch water or waste.

Dr. Hahnemann uses this word in his connotation of
intangible infectious agent to designate the disturbance
causing chronic diseases. He also explains three different
miasma types: psoric, syphilitic and psychotic. These sickly
disorders can and will only be eradicated by the
homeopathic medicine.

Psora (from the Greek psora: scratch, itch) is a skin
disease, particularly, scabies. Psoriasis means to be infected
by psora (obsolete significance). It is a chronic skin disease
in which the skin is covered by an erythema and squamae
(formerly of unknown cause, but some say it is an immune
disease).

In paragraph 81 of the Organon, Hahnemann explains
how the psoric miasma has affected humankind through
inheritance. It is important to mention that Dr. Hahnemann

wrote this text in 1810, and the discoverer of the laws of heritance, the Augustinian monk Gregor Johann Mendel (who was born the same year as Pasteur 1822), published his findings in 1866. These results were unseen until De Vries and other two botany experts rediscovered them in 1900.

Psychosis, from the Greek Sykosis: fig-shaped ulcer, sykon: fig, is a condylomatous disease that cannot be eradicated from the core: Dr. Kent explains this term when he mentions several times the word Sycose; and he refers to the patient as being psychotic.

Finally, syphilis (from Syphilo, character of the poem "De morbo gallico" of Geronimo Fracastor) used to be the most serious venereal disease of all compared in importance to the various types of cancer, and the worst of all diseases: the Acquired Immunodeficiency Syndrome (AIDS). Hahnemann considers this chronic miasma as the deadliest illness of his era.

It is useful for the doctor to know the particular details of the probable cause originating the disease. Equally, the doctor must be aware of the most meaningful features being present in the complete medical history of the chronic disease in order to find and cure the chronic miasma. It is necessary to define the patient state, his/her moral code, intellectuality, profession, habits, life style, social and family relationships, age and sexual activity.

In such a way, the healing power and the remedy and/or drug action will always act out in a centrifugal way, and also, the disease action will do it centripetally. His concept is just about what we think, what we do and what we eat, according to the anthropological and biophysical point of view.

In the Organon (paragraph 78), Samuel Hahnemann states: "chronic diseases are those which agent is a chronic miasma. This chronic miasma and the psora are too deep to be eradicated". The psora (genome acquired through genera- tions) has been able to stipulate distinct morbid shapes being present in millions of people during hundreds of generations, and nowadays we have the responsibility of finding a cure.

Mood and mental states are essential in every disease case whether they are chronic or acute and usually become the starting point about the drug and/or remedy selection. Essays of Personality is all about this; it relates the appropriate drug with the personality and if we do not apply this criterion then the patient will never find relief which is the opposite of our goal.

The order of Essays on Personality, goes from the most sophisticated and complex to the most simple and easiest, all according to my experience which i wanted to share today,

I have observed, as Dr. Hahnemann used to say, in terminally ill patients, that the vital energy working as an entropic state does not exist or is considerably diminished. While measuring medical material and miasmas, I have noticed there is only one positive drug which can help this kind of patients, their personality. This medication allows them to have a respectful death. And this. is something that I also wanted to share with you.

Antonio Ridaura MD.

1 Natrum Muriaticum

Natrum Muriaticum was used by the ancient homeopathic physicians to treat chronic diarrhea. It was also used to cure the ancient diarrhea of the armies (Kent, Materia médica, fourth edition, 1932). A patient being affected by Natrum Muriaticum will, most of the time, suffer from vaginal problems like leucorrhoea and/or candidiasis. There are other types of antidotes such as Plunbum, Thuja and Selenium containing greasy and shiny skin.

Natrum Muriaticum is a deep long-acting treatment. It dominates the body wonderfully and if it is ingested in large doses, it provides enduring changes.

Mental symptoms of this medication originate a long chain: hysterical body and mind structures, crying which substitutes laughing and vice versa; compulsory laughing specially in inappropriate moments; long-acting and spasmodic laughing. Other symptoms: lachrymose, extreme sadness and depression: no matter how happy the situation could be, the patient is not able to get encouraged. He is caged thinking about all his/her impressions. The patient gets easily distressed and due to trivial issues starts to remember every unpleasant thing so that he can continue being affected by sorrow. Any type of comforting deteriorates the patient's state of mind. Melancholy: the patient becomes tearful but suddenly becomes angry; the patient represents to want some of affection but gets mad as soon he feels it. The patient experiences headaches: he walks erratically from side to side, forgets everything very easily, is unable to calculate, unable to meditate, finds difficult to remember what he was going to say, gets distracted while reading or listening. The mind collapse is very profound.

Pain pierces like electroshocks: convulsive shaking of the limbs while sleeping, spasms and brief— transparent pain. The patient is hypersensitive to anything and gets emotional and excited without difficulty. Pain can occur if the patient is exposed to heated environment and it gets worse staying indoors. For this reason and in order to find relief, it is better to take some fresh air. Having sweated, the patient gets a cold regularly though being outdoors

Skin appears waxy and hydropic. Noticeable emaciation and skin is dry, withered and wrinkled: a kid might seem like an old man. This apparent affliction diminishes

from the face as soon as the patient improves. This emaciation occurs from the top-down; the patient neck bones become apparent which makes him look bony; but hips and lower limbs continue to be plump and voluptuous. Also, Lypocodium Clavatum (Which will be discussed later on) has top-down emaciation as well. Different remedies help us differentiate one from the other.

Mucous membranes outstanding secretion is aqueous or really dense and whitish just as an egg white. Coryza is prominent and even it contains aqueous secretion, the natural construction is full of whitish dense postules; the patient expels dense and whitish mucus during morning. There is glutinous oozing in the eyes and the ears produce a whitish dense glutinous discharge. Whitish leucorrhea is dense as well. When it comes to gonorrhea, infection has been there for a long time and has become blennorheic; urethra turns acutely itchy after urinating.

Headaches are intense; head appears as if it were to explode or that it is being compressed. These pains are accompanied by hammering and pounding sensations; when one starts walking, the headache becomes an acute hammering pain. Hammering-like pains when waking up in the morning and pain that appears during the final stage of sleeping. During the first stage of the night, there is a high level of restlessness; the patient goes to bed really late and wakes up with a hammering pain in the head. There is also the presence of headaches that start between 10:00 to 11:00 AM and last until 3:00 PM, sometimes they even last until the evening.

Stomach and liver are closely related. Stomach is swollen due to the presence of gas. After eating, there is a lump in the stomach: it appears as if the meal requires a long time to be digested and this worsens by eating. Vomiting of whitish dense mucous provides comfort. There is a severe sense of thirstiness that cannot be fulfilled. In the liver region we find pounding and ripping pain. Intestines are swollen due to gas. There is a tendency to lack of activity of all intestinal functions, defecation is difficult and when it does take place there are hard lumps. The bladder also is prone to a lack of activity: patient has to wait in order for the urine stream to come out and it does so in a slow manner as a few droplets flowing with very low pressure. After urination, there is a feeling that more urine is about to come out. Patient is unable to urinate if someone is present. There is a constant and frequent urge to urinate.

Natrum Muriaticum patients suffer from severe stomach disease and are voracious eaters. Skin symptoms tend to be very noticeable: skin appears to be transparent, waxy, greasy, and shiny.

Shivers appear in the morning at 10:30 AM every day. Every three to four days. They start at the limbs which turn blue. There is a pulsating pain in the head, face is constipated. Sometimes becomes delirious and talks about anything. There is constant maniac activity. These symptoms escalate all the way to a constipated state. There is the presence of thirstiness and the need to drink cold water during the attack. During the coldness period, the patient cannot improve when exposed to heat or when covered up. He requires cold drinks.

We might naturally suppose that a person that is freezing to death should require heat but a Natrum Muriaticum patient cannot stand heat. Teeth chatter and the patient appears restless pacing back and forth, bones hurt as if they were going to break and there is vomiting under constipated conditions. During the presence of fever, the patient is so hot that his fingers are almost on fire due to the intense heat and he falls asleep in a constipated sleep or stupor. Sweating alleviates this condition: generalized pain decreases due to perspiration and cephalalgia disappears with time. Shivering, fever, and perspiration are intense.

Natrum Muriaticum is useful for mothers, after delivery when unable to recover. Mothers are weak and easily excitable; the presence of lochia is extended, profuse and whitish. Hair from head and genitals is lost. Milk production stops or the child does not want it. It is useful in post-partum pain when there is a sub-involution of the uterus and when it is in an extended congestive state. The patient is highly affected by noise, music, or door slamming. Craves salt, and feels an aversion towards bread, wine, and substantial meals. Sour wine upsets her stomach.

Natrum Muriaticum will heal the symptoms and will trigger the production of milk.

The Natrum Muriaticum Personality

- Natrum Muriaticum patients cry easily or become upset at the slightest motivation
- The first thing they do is look at their reflection in the mirror
- Frequently wake up in a foul mood
- Sleep is very light and not very deep, almost any noise will cause them to wake up and it is not easy for them to fall asleep
- Are jealous, possessive, irritable, and resentful
- Become upset at the slightest motivation
- Are almost never mistaken
- It is very difficult for them to ask for forgiveness
- Are very direct in their judgments
- Are pathological liars, not very affectionate, are loving only when they feel like it, almost always suffer from gynecological problems (leucorrhea, candidiasis, moniliasis, etc)
- When they work, they would rather be at work where they spends most of the useful part of the day
- When they stay at home, they are obsessive with regards to cleanliness
- They are very detail oriented, similar to an Arsenicum Album patient (notice even the slightest possible detail)
- If she is a wife or girlfriend, she is very inexpressive, and only when she feels like it and not when she is provoked
- A Natrum Muriaticum patient has noticeable facial lines, grays prematurely
- Is very affected when offended
- Possessive, jealous, resentful, and a pathological liar
- Always wants to be a leader and stand out
- If a door closes, they will open twenty
- Are always thinking
- It is the personality where you make the most of intellectual capacity

- They reason about all that they want, and they always come out triumphant
- Every enterprise he undertakes will flourish
- A prodigious memory
- They never forget important dates, facts, or information
- They see a pleasure in reading whether they are men or women

2 Phosphorous

A chronic flu and swelling. A dry burning sensation and heartburn in the stomach. Cramps. Bloody vomit. Discomfort and constipation in the pit of the stomach (cardias). Chronic diarrhea (especially in small children) in tuberculosis and typhoid fever. Bloody urine. A chronic hoarse voice, a persistent flu, larynx and pharynx ailments. Lung and pharynx tuberculosis. Coughing with bloody expectoration. Swelling of the lungs. Bronchitis (especially in small children). Asthma. Heart disease. Blood spotting disease. Scurvy. Paralysis.

Phosphorous suffers from burping, especially after eating. Usually has an unsuccessful urge to vomit and an increase of acid levels or the taste of whatever he has ingested remains. A dry sour burning taste in the mouth and the esophagus. There is a canine hunger. Discomfort due to worms after eating, heartburn, drowsiness, heat and insufficient breathing. There is nausea, especially in the morning, at night, and after having eaten. There is vomiting of whatever has been ingested. There is the presence of bile, mucus, and blood (any ailment of the esophagus that produces pathologies such as ulcers or varicose veins in the stomach).

There are plethora and stomachaches, especially to the touch, and after eating. There is a burning sensation in the pit of the stomach during swallowing, as if the food could not go through and would go back up. The belly is elevated, especially after eating. There is a confinement of gas and diarrhea along with sharp pains in the stomach area, especially when in bed. Soft abdomen for a long time.

There is a difficulty to defecate and there is blood and mucus when doing so. Excrement has a gray, black or greenish appearance that are also undigested and involuntary with subsequent depression. There is a secretion of mucus from the anus that is always open. There are hemorrhoids that bleed easily. There is the presence of blood in the urine with many sediments leaving a thin film.

There is a rebellious hoarse voice, as well as a disappearance of the voice. There is also a dryness in larynx and pharynx. A cough that is caused by beating pulses and an itching in neck and chest, especially during the night. There is a dry and uncomfortable cough, caused by cold air, drinks, and discourse, as well as due to speaking in public. There is a cough with saline pus expectoration, especially in the morning and afternoon. There is dense or striated mucus that is bloody or that is pure blood.

A constipated heaviness and plethora in the chest. Sharp pains on the sides of the chest (chronic obstructive pulmonary disease). It feels as if being wounded or hurt in the chest. There is a.heavy and difficult breathing especially during the afternoon or in the morning, with a feeling of suffocation during the night. There is a noisy breathing, as if the air were full of liquid. There is mucus especially when the patient is lying down or asleep. There are heart palpitations especially after eating in the morning or in the afternoon, as well as when sitting. When there is a moral affliction, the patient cannot bear to be on his side.

There is spotting of the skin that can also be marble–like and large or small spots that are blood—like (erysipelas). When they suffer from any type of injury, they bleed more than usual. Gums are swollen and bleed easily. There is nose bleeding, bloody vomiting or expectoration, and defecation with blood. Blood appears to precipitate and wind strongly down the veins.

There is a great weakness and sometimes a sudden depression. There is a nervous weakening with heaviness of the limbs that sometimes get numb or paralyzed. There is a paralyzing of one limb or the other and numbness. There is a shaking due to the slightest of efforts.

They are very sensitive to catching a cold when outdoors, especially in cool weather. There are pains accompanying all types of atmospheric variations. Almost every ailment appears during the night or early in the morning, when in bed, as well as after eating. There is a scary or afraid state of mind, especially when the patient is left alone, when there is rainy weather, and in the afternoon.

The Phosphorous Personality

- Are confident, expressive and friendly
- Often make friends and are not resentful
- Very optimistic
- Love to be the center of all attention
- Have a talent for drawing
- As children, they are restless, nervous, and affectionate
- Are afraid of the dark
- Imaginative
- Love having company, being popular
- Blush easily
- Hate tests or homework
- Have well—defined traits
- Are almost completely bald as adults
- Never suffer from varicose alterations
- Do not like being alone, they are shy, very emotional and nostalgic
- When they get angry, they really get angry
- Are creative: they love drawing, painting and modeling
- Are easily offended
- Are very sensitive, apathetic and restless
- Are excellent observers and very loving
- Are always ready to help others
- They are sometimes critical in a crude way
- Are more than human
- Are almost always diffuse
- Sometimes have big appetites

3 Sepia Oficinalis

Headaches with blood accumulation, in pregnant women as well. Chronic cephalalgia, swelling of the skull, with convulsive movements in the head, all the way to the back or to the front. A pain in the face. Stomach flu and cramps. Vomiting, especially also in pregnant women. Liver disease. Abdominal plethora, loose or flapping belly, prominent and hard belly (also in multiparous women). Hard belly, constipated. Hemorrhoidal pain. Dysmenorrhea, leucorrhea. Abortions. A drop of the uterus or of the clitoris.

Sudden dizziness and head problems are present, when outdoors, when writing, or when waking up early. Violent headaches with nausea and vomiting when the head is moved, especially in the morning, when waking up, or just on one side, as if the head were to explode. This occurs especially at night, after going to bed, or when waking up. Throbbing headaches are acute or with a hammering sensation, and with an important blood flow to the head, convulsive pain in the head and facial bones. There is an appearance of scattered dark yellow spots on face, nose, or cheeks, with a difficulty to open eyes and the presence of a darkened vision.

A great speed or aversion towards food, and there is the presence of heartburn, gas, soreness or burning sensation in the neck, beating in the stomach region, hiccups, burning or heating sensation, rapid heartbeats, nausea, vomiting and acceleration in the movement, headaches, stomachaches. Stomach and belly are swollen, a pain due to a feeling of emptiness in the stomach. There is a sense of heaviness and pressure in the belly, which is hard and prominent as if it were to explode; along with a presence of acute or swelling stomachaches, especially when moving or at night, with a great urge to defecate. There are sharp pains in the liver region, a great urge to defecate, with unsuccessful or insufficient results in a slow manner; with ball-shaped excrement with mucus or blood. There is a drop of the intestines with a burning, itching sensation. There is a constriction of the urine stream with pain and burning in the urethra. There is a precocious, insufficient or suppressed menstruation; a foul secretion from the clitoris or mucous or yellowish or greenish red secretion, or pus; as well as a burning sensation with eczema or abrasion of the area.

Pain decreases with strenuous exercise and increases when resting in the afternoon and at night, constipation pain in the lower abdomen, a gestational pain as a consequence of suppressing sweat in feet, of the suppression of menstruation at a critical age; irregularities in venous flow. There is yellow, gray, or liver-colored spotting of the skin, especially on the face, chest, or stomach region. This is especially present in irritable-tempered and easily excited people who are prone to sadness, anguishing concerns and health issues. They cry easily and are prone to heartache to the point of becoming fed up with life. There is a misanthropic irritability and bad temper, together with a weak memory.

The Sepia Oficinalis Personality

- Irritable; always have a taste for fast food or snacks
- If they are women, they almost always wear pants
- Have sunken eyes, yellowish or sallow skin
- Have a taste for dance, or folk dancing
- Dark eyes, are usually slim
- Very sensitive to climate changes, everything affects them
- Get easily tired, are indifferent and try to avoid other people
- Cry for no reason
- Their tongue is clean during their period, and are sexually unstable
- Are afraid of poverty, hypochondriac, and pessimistic
- Are afraid of their future and of death
- When they work and they like it, they are very dedicated
- They are pathological liars, have a varying temper, sardonic
- Before getting their periods, they do not feel well, and feel worse when they get it
- Are irate, and get easily angered. They do not like to be contradicted
- Are not very gregarious, not very affectionate towards others. if she is a daughter, towards parents or siblings, if she is married towards husband or children
- Always have problems of face spotting or acne, especially in the nasolabial region
- Have very expressive face or features, sunken, unexpressive eyes; and are sometimes very unbearable

4 Silicea Terra

It is an adequate remedy to treat those ailments that develop slowly, in certain periods of the year, and under specific circumstances. A Silicea Terra patient really feels the cold and his symptoms develop with time and cold weather. Symptoms appear after taking a shower. Silicea Terra is under a state of weakness, confusion, fear, and defeated. If the description of such state were to be heard from a prominent preacher, an attorney,.or by a confident person (confident about his thoughts and character when speaking in public), he would talk about reaching a state in which he is afraid of speaking in public, where he is so concerned about himself that he cannot concentrate on the topic, that he is afraid of failure and his mind becoming blank. He is burnout due to extended mental strain. He will always say that when he is able to overcome himself and control the situation can act adequately. His confidence returns and performs in such a way that he is able to fulfill his activities in a quick and confident manner.

The peculiar state of Silicea Terra lies in the fear of failure. The patient is confronted with an activity he has to fulfill that is out of the ordinaiy; he is then afraid to fail despite conducting the activity adequately. The primary stages are such that the time might come in which he will be unable to perform his activities efficiently. He will still require the Silicea Terra medication.

This medication is not adequate for irritability and nervous strain that follow mental fatigue of businessmen but it is good to treat mental fatigue of professionals: attorneys, students, priests. An attorney can say: "I have never been the same after that".

There is the appearance of warts on skin, wet eruptions, pimples, blisters, abscesses, and oozing cavities. Silicea Terra cures oozing cavities with hardened ridges. There is a flowing discharge, copious mucous secretions of eyes, nose, ears, breast, and vagina. Discomfort related to the suppression of discharge and perspiration. Such suppressions cause a certain state in the body that threaten the little order that might be left. A foul smelling perspiration of the feet after having had the feet wet, this is followed by shivering and violent discomfort. SiliceaTerra cures sweaty feet when the symptoms apply or the discomfort persists since the suppression of the sweat in feet. There is dense yellowish discharge. Patients say: "I have had this discharge for many years". When this statement is investigated, it is found that there has been a certain commotion, some sort of cooling that suppressed the sweat in feet that has not reappeared since then.

Silicea Terra will bring back the sweat in feet, it will make the flowing discharge disappear and in due time will cure sweaty feet. Flowing discharge of the nose and other points; indurations, tumors, chronic gastritis, brain burnout, all related to the suppression of some sort of sweat in feet, otorrhea, or the elimination of a blister.

Patient suffers from dizziness to the point of fainting, with the presence of nausea. There is a vertigo that goes up the spinal cord. There are headaches that worsen with mental strain, excessive studying, noise, movement, and even due to the vibration caused by footsteps, light, leaning forward, for making an effort to defecate, to take; because of cold air, and all types of contact. There are scaly, wet, eruptions on the scalp, eczema, or capitis.

Silicea Terra is adequate for phagedenic ulcers caused by syphilis. Those ulcers that undermine and extend to the pericranium, for inflammatory ailments between the scalp and the skull, for developing tumors filled with dense' liquid. This remedy will eliminate blood tumors, even in children. Cephalotoma neonatum, encondroma. Silicea Terra is especially useful to treat cartilage ailments, the growth around joints and in fingers, hands, and feet.

Silicea Terra ailments are related to hardened glands, but especially those around the neck and cervical, salivary, and above all parotid glands that are swollen and hardened. Parotid glands become hypertrophic and hardened, as a result of being exposed to cold. Silicea Terra is recommended for the treatment of the most chronic forms, due to the profound psora.

This, along with a large amount of eye swelling and ailments, ulcerations of the cornea, eyelid blisters, burning discharge in the palpebral margins, reddening of the face; photophobia with eye discomfort, watery fluid discharge that is copious, bloody, dense and yellow, syphilitic iritis, oozing and piercing blisters of the cornea, spots and scarring; eyes swollen due to trauma, palpebral tumors, tear conduct narrowing or fistulae.

The complexion of a Silicea Terra patient is silky, waxy, anemic, and tired. There are pustular and vesicular eruptions all over the face. Nostrils are swollen and lips are cracked. There is also the formation of scabs and hardened areas on the skin. The tendency is that soft tissue becomes hardened, and hard tissue becomes keratinized. Teeth become decayed and enamel is lost. Just as Silicea Terra is present as a component of bones, teeth, and especially dentine, they are also composed of calcium silicate. A Silicea Terra patient has teeth that are rough and have lost their brightness. Tooth decay appears easily and many times reach the ridges of the dental alveoli. Teeth hurt when temperature changes. They become yellow, gums tend to retract, and teeth start to come out or easily move (paradontosis). There are serious parodental problems, such as severe abscesses. The pain caused by these abscesses improves with heat. The tongue is swollen (almost filling the entire mouth cavity) ripping pain that becomes worse at night.

There is adenitis in the throat that reaches the neck causing severe pain. There is also a severe hypertrophy of the tonsils that can even cause suppuration. There might also be abscesses present in the parotid glands along with an almost frequent suppuration. The condition of the patient condition worsens when exposed to cold, and improves with heat.

A Silicea Terra patient will suffer from digestive problems due to nausea and vomiting and at the same time, this can affect part of the hepatic region. He has an aversion towards hot meals and craves cold food. His food and everything he ingests needs to be less than lukewarm. He likes cold water and ice cream.

Extreme heat and cold can easily affect a Silicea Terra patient who dislikes milk, and many times breast milk will induce vomiting and diarrhea. He suffers from stomachaches and severe abdominal pain. Pressure worsens, there are flatulent cramps and he has a feeling of bruising. Pain improves with heat and when eating. There is constipation present and when the patient is able to defecate, he does so sweating and in the shape of small balls.

Silicea Terra is one of the great remedies to cure nasal flu and tuberculoid infiltrations. Therefore, we find hydrosalpingitis and pio—salpingitis in women, amenorrhea that lasts for months; waxy cysts in the vagina that are the size of a grain of rice and can grow to the size of an orange. The patient also suffers from excoriating leucorrhea with pain and can also have mastitis.

The patient has a cough, in the first stages of tuberculosis or pneumonia; wet asthma and rasping breath. The patient is pale, with a waxy appearance, anemic, with a noticeable deep depression and a terrible thirst.

Silicea Terra has abundant, fetid, greenish and purulent expectoration during the day. Has a chronic tendency to colds that fix in the chest with dyspnea that can escalate to a chronic bronchitis.

Silicea Terra adapts especially to pneumonia and chronic bronchopulmonary problems. The hands and feet of Silicea Terra sweat profusely.

The Silicea Terra Personality

- A tenacious, obsessed, friendly, and sensitive person
- Lack of confidence, hesitating when it comes to beginning new tasks
- When they concentrate on a task ofjob they are very obsessed and finish it, despite hunger or tiredness to the point of exhaustion
- They are very careful with the slightest of details
- When they get to a place, they have to recognize, check, and determine if they like it. If they are not aware or comfortable, they just leave
- Shy, lack confidence, and are afraid of failure
- They are afraid of starting newjobs or tasks that they might not like, but when they do like it, they work very hard
- They fear for their health and their future
- They are very sensitive or resentful for something that is not worth it
- Extremely perfectionist, obsessed, and very impatient
- They sometimes become enraged and are easily offended
- They are usually very shy, in order to reach a decision they think very hard about it, and are not direct in theirjudgments
- Once they are sure and they like what they are doing, they are very detail oriented and careful
- When they are children, they have developmental problems. They are weak, easily affected by cold, and diaphoretic
- Usually, sweaty hands are a classical symptom of this personality that is sometimes so severe that hands can be soaked in sweat
- They are good at observing, and have shy eyes and face
- Are extremely concerned about saving
- They are usually long-lined

- As children, they are different to other personalities, because they have different heights, big heads, and noticeable bellies
- Skin suppurates easily, breakable nails and hyper sensible skin

5 Nux Vomica

Head heaviness, vertigo. Headache: dizziness, especially after restless and sleepless nights, mental efforts due to excess of wine or coffee. Hysterical women and people that never leave the room or their own room. Face pain, toothache. Cold—related swollen neck. Chronic stomach flu, chronic cramps in stomach (especially in coffee lovers.) Chronic nausea or vomiting (especially in pregnant women and men that get usually drunk.) Compulsive delirium tremens, burping and hiccups. Menstrual cramps. Pain and discomfort. Flatulence, hernia pain. Swelling and constipation. Hysterical and hypochondriac, convulsion, paralysis, apoplexy. Hard constipated stomach (especially in pregnant women and those who never leave the room). Hemorrhoid pain. Pain when urinating. Pain related to position changed or prolapsed uterus. Cough. Influenza. Cold. Asthma. Heart palpitations (especially in ailments caused by flatulence after irritation in a nervous person who suffers from gastralgia.) Sporadic fever (with gastric symptoms.)

The patient suffers from head heaviness, confused mind that does not allow thinking nor picking up thoughts especially during the morning while waking up, just as if one has not slept enough. Vertigo and hung over feeling that increases after meals due to movement, when leaning forward and meditating. Pain on the side of the head or as if carrying a nail stuck in the skull, also accompanied by nausea and vomiting. Periodic headache, with blood flow towards the head. Uncomfortable sight sensibility, noise and tremor in the brain when walking. Sensibility in the scalp, especially when touching it. Rheumatic pain on the face, especially on cheeks, accompanied by swelling. Compulsive movements of face muscles. Toothache that extends up to the upper part of the head and it is caused by the outdoors, coffee and wine, which is increased when drinking cold water or something else, and decreased by heat. Teeth move from their alveoli.

Neck pain when swallowing with slightly red and swollen palate and as if the patient had a foreign object in it. Unpleasant taste in mouth particularly when waking up and after eating. Repulsiveness caused by all foods, even bread, coffee and smoking.

After eating, the patient feels a series of ailments; he mainly feels the stomach, a swollen hypochondrium and abdomen, depression, confused head, drowsiness, hiccups, burps, nausea and vomiting what has been eaten or unsuccessful attempts to vomit, particularly in the morning.

Fullness and pressure in the stomach, mainly after eating. Stomachache, painful contraction due to constipation, when fasting or after eating. Thus, sensibility and excessive stomach hardening. Stone-|ike heaviness, especially in the upper and lower part of the stomach, as if suffering from cramps caused from flatulence, resulting in hernias. Efforts and an urgent need to stool.

Difficult and tough bowel movement, often with blood marks. Chronic belly constipation, lumpiness in the anal veins. Need to urinate with scarce urine; urine retention. Pain in the stomach, bearing down, pain in the back and spine-making difficult to stand straight, to walk and to lean forward; difficulty to have bowel movement. Menstrual period appears ahead of time or too heavy.

Cold-related hoarseness, dry and rough throat. Cough that increases with movement and when speaking, as well as through the night and morning. Dry interrupted cough, headache, as if the head were to blast, accompanied by pain from shaking in chest and stomach, especially after going to bed. Compulsive cough, as if neck were stretched, closed throat and chest particularly at night when the patient is lying down. Suffocation attacks with palpitation after midnight. Chest convulsions, mainly after a nervous irritation.

Cold and chills without being noticeably cold, followed by extreme heat, thirst and sweating and extreme headache, great depression, ----stomach and nausea, occurring during the periods of fever, slow bowel movement, flatulence and swollen stomach. Fever in the morning with slight cold, followed by extreme heat and thirst. Backache when cold ascends. Shivering even with the slightest movements, even if the patient is in bed and in spite of the heat and sweating.

Especially in the early morning or after walking, there is excessive irritability of nervous system and sensitivity or susceptibility of all senses with immediate depression, as well as heaviness and trembling of the limbs, especially early in the morning or after walking. Avoids movement and outdoors, tends to be moody, easily gets scared or anguished. Overtiredness of the head after mental work. Vertigo attacks especially in the mornings, after meals, in the afternoon or in bed. He may feel dazed, or have convulsions of particular muscles or entire limb; numbness, deafness, paralyzed legs or arms with a cold sensation. There is little stability, leg and knee shaking, as well as sudden weakness and shaking.

Pains and ailments increase almost always in the mornings, after waking up, or after meals as well as after having coffee or after mental work. There are pains caused by being seated for a long period of time, lack of movement or air, in which case a noticeable improvement is shown. He gets constipation and the flu easily, as well as all the flu related symptoms. There are aches resulting form mental work, getting upset, alcohol, coffee or tobacco intake.

The patient wakes up very early, without being able to fall back to sleep, he is moody and has an uncomfortable feeling of not having enough sleep, all the more if there is dryness or body thinness. People of dark skin and hair are more likely to get hemorrhoids and plethora of the lower stomach.

Nux Vomica Personality

- Irritable, leader and long-lineal
- If women, slender or Barbie type body
- Gets upset when questioned or in conversations
- Mentally active
- Enjoys doing things on her own and being self—sufficient
- Easily cries, needs lots of affection
- Fears failure and tries to protect her future
- Hypochondriac
- Gets angry and infuriates when interrupted
- Confident, jealous and loving
- Supports others decisions is a born leader
- If he is a student, he is followed by his classmates
- He has serious digestive problems
- Is very possessive, obsessively critical, direct in his judgments, dreamer
- Is specific and direct for decision making
- Competes with himself, meticulous
- Is decisive in any work he carries out
- Is determined and expressive
- Very organized in every enterprise he pursues
- Is a great friend
- Defends his and other's concepts if he agrees
- If he fails in an enterprise, he quickly recovers and succeeds, even if it takes some time
- They are usually thin children
- He is has a very expressive look and immediately detect whether they want something or not

6 Pulsatilla Nigricans

This medication is said to be adequate for blonde patients, especially for weeping blonde patients. It is a polychrest and it is also one of the most used remedies and of the most frequently abused, too.

The typical patient of Pulsatilla Nigricans is a young lady prone to crying. If judged by her aspect, she seems plethoric and healthy, nevertheless she is quite nervous, restless, versatile, docile, and can be easily persuaded. She is sweet, kind, and very prone to shed tears, but she is extremely irritable as well, not in the sense of being a brawler, but of getting angry easily.

She is extremely sensitive. She tends to feel or fears to be unappreciated and she is very sensitive to a social influence. There is melancholy, sadness, wailing, and despair within her. She is mainly religious, fanatic, imaginative, full of opinions and whimsies, and extremely excitable. She tends to imagine that cultivating the company of the opposite sex is dangerous and that incurring in acts that society admits to be good for the human species is also dangerous, being these capricious concepts related to food or behavior; for example, she considers that drinking milk is not good, therefore she abstains from it. She considers that certain food products are not good for the human kind. Her aversion to marriage is a very noticeable symptom. A man can get into his head that it is noxious to have sexual relations with his wife and he will therefore abstain from it.

He has religious extravagances and a very pronounced tendency to adjust his behavior to religious concepts. He has fixed ideas concerning the Bible, which he has misunderstood and what is worse, uses them for his own harm. He walks the road to sanctity until he becomes an insane fanatic. He considers he is in a beatific mental state or otherwise, that he is out of grace because of his sins. This condition progresses until he becomes insane in other aspects and then, he remains sitting, taciturn all day, day after day. He will not answer questions unless he is under pressure, and he will only answer "yes" or "no" or simply by moving his head. Puerperal insanity in a woman who has been sweet, kind, and prone to shed tears, later on she becomes sad and taciturn to the point that she remains sat in a chair the entire day, only answering with head movements.'

Many ailments are related to stomach feebleness, indigestion, or menstrual disorders. Women with such aches tend to undergo abortions; they have irregular menstruations, and false pregnancies. Mental symptoms are often associated to uterine and ovarian disorders.

Along with such mental state, the state of the organism worsens if the room temperature is hot and improves with movement. She is tearful, sad, and discouraged, but feels better by walking outdoors, particularly if the day is cold and invigorating and the atmosphere is clear and fresh. In a warm room she feels suffocated, her ailments increase and she may even feel a nervous coldness if she transpires due to the heat in the room.

Inflammatory symptoms (neuralgias and rheumatisms) ease with cold weather, by eating and drinking cold things, and by applying cold things on the skin, even in the hands if they are cold. Cold drinks relieve, even when the patient is not thirsty. Cold food is well digested, but warm food causes the body to heat up, worsening the symptoms. Ice cold water relieves as it descends through the esophagus and the stomach retains it, even though there is no thirst.

Vein widening is produced, which is why in this patient ulcers surrounded by varicose veins are usual. Ulcers that emit black blood which, at first forms little black blood clots; blood emission is not abundant, and so it forms clots easily. Formation of blood clots similar to coal tar, dark and fetid. The ulcers bleed and exude a waterish, bloody fluid that can be very thick, yellowish or greenish sometimes.

The typical patient of Pulsatilla Nigricans suffers from violent cephaleas, young ladies tend to have strong headaches when their menstruation is upcoming. Such headaches are associated to suppressed menstruations or other menstrual disorders; headaches are not originated by such disorders but are associated to them. Aches around the temple and the sides of the head are frequent in the patient of Pulsatilla Nigricans. Before the headaches start, during or after the menstruation (but more often before the menstruation), certain state of general congestion, ecstasy, and vein tumefaction prevails and the relief of the cephalea is produced when the menstruation begins if the menstruation flow is normal; in these cases, nervous and cephalic symptoms are common. If the flux is scarce, often a little less than leucorrhoea, only a small clot of black blood is produced during a whole day. Unilateral cephaleas and other unilateral ailments are characteristic in Pulsatilla Nigricans patients: transpiration in one side of the face or the head, fever in one side of the body; one side is fresh and normal and the other one is heated. I remember a case of puerperal fever with transpiration in one side of the body, dry heat in the other, and confusion of the remaining symptoms; Pulsatilla Nigricans was administrated and the patient healed.

The type of headache of the Pulsatilla Nigricans patient is congestive and palpitating; plenty of pain in the head which is relieved by cold applications, external pressure and, sometimes, slow movements in the outdoors. It worsens when lying down at rest; it intensifies at nightfall and increases gradually during the night, worsening when moving the eyes and leaning over; such aches tend to be constrictive, palpitating and congestive. Other common symptoms are headaches accompanied by periodical nausea and vomits with sour breath. Headaches caused by eating excessively; even though the patient longs for an ice cream, headache and congestion return after eating it.

As for the eyes, she suffers from catarrhal symptoms; pustules in the eyelids and the eyeball, acute inflammations, thick yellow–green pus on the cornea, and granular eyelids.

Loss of the smell sense happens with acute and chronic colds: during the night there is much nasal obstruction. During the day, the patient blows her nose, but by sundown it gets blocked and it is no longer possible to clean it off. It is important to remember that mental symptoms worsen at night. In the morning, the patient wakes up with a blocked nose, but she can clean it off. She has bitter taste in the mouth and the tongue is dirty, so she needs to brush her teeth thoroughly and use mouthwash before having breakfast. Therefore, it is noticeable that mouth and stomach symptoms are worse in the morning, while mental symptoms are worse at night, with nasal obstructions being present as well.

Compare this symptomatology with cough: in Pulsatilla Nigricans patients, cough is dry at nights, with some production of fluid, in the morning with no abundant expectoration. During the night, there is a sensation of severe, dry constriction. This obstruction causes breathing difficulty. Hence, we can conclude that the Pulsatilla

Nigricans patient suffers from recurrent and inveterate colds with loss of the sense of smell and thick yellowish septum, showing improvement outdoors if the patient is nervous, shy and condescending, whose nose gets obstructed at nights but has abundant flow in the mornings.

Frequently, acute colds present nasal hemorrhage caused by blowing the nose, besides, the nose bleeds easily, so is subject to epistaxis.

Pulsatilla Nigricans is very useful for hay fever; a considerable study is required for its treatment, which is why it is important to deal with the previous concepts of the patient, which bother him and will make him refuse to be subject of study. The patient may want his hay fever to be treated, but he refuses to talk, does not want to be asked about his hemorrhoids, thickened skin on the sole, and his pain in the sacrum or about diarrhea, which alternates with constipation. These symptoms ameliorate when hay fever is present. Sometimes the patient will say that he is always fine, except when he suffers from hay fever; he may feel fine, but it is impossible that he is actually fine. He has always suffered from this ailments and he will not allow to be bothered with questions about such condition. Hay fever alone will hardly provide enough indications to prescribe a remedy.

Pulsatilla Nigricans patients have symptoms and prolapse. When hay fever is present, every other symptom ameliorates, this is why the patient is only conscious of the fever, but all the symptoms are interrelated. In Naturum Muriaticum patients, the symptoms will be worse in the morning and towards noon; however, in Pulsatilla Nigricans patients the symptoms will be worse at night: the nose fills up with thick, sticky, yellow—green mucus and when the nose is finally cleared up, the burning sensation of dryness and itching will prevail. If room remains warm at night, the patient will not be able to sleep; the Naturum Muriaticum is somewhat similar in this aspect with regard to the itching and the impossibility to sleep in a warm room. Release can continue day and night in Naturum Muriaticum patients as well.

There is a sickish, mottled appearance in the face, it is often livid, blended with yellow and other colors which denote poor health. There might be swelling of the veins, plethoric sensation; a colored face that seems to be normal, which is why the patient will hardly be distressed about it. Other symptoms include suffocation and color rushes in the face, which can also seem sunken; erysipelas that itch and burn may appear in the face sometimes, spreading to the scalp. Facial skin tends to be oversensitive to touch.

Mumps and parotid glands inflammation: if a woman suffering from mumps gets cold, her breasts will swell up caused by mammary glands inflammation. In young ladies who have had cold drinks, the parotid gland inflammation will decrease very soon and the corresponding mammary gland will be swollen; sometimes both breasts, and sometimes, inflammation begins in one breast and follows to the other. In men, the testicle gets swollen. Pulsatilla Nigricans is one of the most important remedies for this kind of metastasis, where spreading ailments emerge. Pulsatilla Nigricans is the remedy used generally in case of extremely swollen testicles on boys suffering from mumps. Carbo vegetabilis is another good remedy, but it must only be administered to patients that fit into this classification. Abrotanum is also used when there are migrating symptoms, such as the Pulsatilla Nigricans patient has. For example, rheumatism migrating from one articulation to another, erratic neurological affections, and inflammation migrating from one articulation to another. However, there is something distinctive about them: Pulsatilla Nigricans keeps its own texture and when it moves to any other point, it does not change or assume a different illness appearance. Abrotanum, in the other hand, has the same metastasis but provokes diagnostic changes and the allopath says "This is a different illness." The patient has diarrhea today, and if he suppresses it due to stubbornness, causing inflammatory rheumatism, which may be considered as a new illness. Suppression of diarrhea, any hemorrhage, or the extirpation of hemorrhoids provokes excrescence somewhere else. If a summer ailment is suppressed in the case of a boy, he will present hepatic or neurological symptoms, or marasmus with emaciation that will spread from bottom to top.

Many ailments seem to manifest on the lower abdomen: inflammation, distension, flatulence, colic pain, borborygmus, food fermentation, menstruation disorders or diarrhea. There is a plenty of painful sensitivity and tumefaction. Full abdomen, stomach and pelvic organs are sensitive to palpitations. There is distension after eating, particularly when the food was greasy and nourishing;vein plethora and generalized venous plethora. It provokes some sort of abdominal tumid repletion, certain fullness sensation, which is why she needs to wear loose dresses or to lay down, because she is so swollen. Associated with the abdominal dilatation, face and lips are swollen and bloated, the eyes are red and the feet are so swollen she cannot wear shoes. Thus, there is a sensation of descending traction and great feebleness which is usually associated to menstrual or uterine disorders; that sensation of descending traction is known as prolapsed uterus and it is felt throughout the abdomen. The prolapsed uterus is also described as a funnel sensation, as if the organs struggled to get out; it is a real descending traction. Extreme sensitivity in the abdomen, particularly in the lower part; the patient cannot be standing for a long period of time; neither can she walk too much due to the weight she feels and the descending traction. Labor-like pains in the back and uterus; it appears that the menstruation is going to begin, and it is common that the Pulsatilla Nigricans patient feels about to menstruate the entire month.

Abdominal and intestinal symptoms are related: sharp, migrating and pains; pains that provoke vomit, stomach cramps associated to dysentery and diarrhea; watery or greenish depositions.

Frequent and scarce micturition; the need to urinate is urgent. There is plenty of extremely painful tenesmus; sanguinolent, burning and itchy urine; even when there is barely a drop of urine in the bladder, the patient feels the urgent need to urinate. The patient cannot lie down on her back without feeling the need to urinate. She may sleep through the entire night if she avoids resting on her back, but the moment she does rest on her back, she will feel that if she does not hurry, the urine will irresistibly flow. The patient has involuntary micturitions when she coughs, laughs or sneezes, because of a sudden allergy or the noise of a door slam. Pulsatilla Nigricans patients have urine leaks caused by the slightest provocation, and have to make a mental effort to retain it; when they prepare to sleep, the urine flows. Enthusiastic, little, sweet, kind, fresh, and plethoric young ladies which have to kick out their sheets at night, suffer from nocturnal enuresis. if the young lady has yellowish, sallow skin, she is sickish and looses urine during the first dream, she needs <u>Sepia Oficinalis</u>.

Loosing urine during the first dream is considered as an outstanding symptom, but it may be caused by the patients effort: if she has been retaining the urine during the day, it is common that she loses it during the first dream, when the mind is unconscious. <u>Causticum</u> and Sepia Oficinalis are commonly used remedies for cases of involuntary micturition during the first dream. I, however, have achieved success treating this condition with many other remedies; for example, in the case of a middle-aged male who flooded his bed as soon as he fell asleep at night. There are only few remedies to these symptoms, and he had already taken all of them, so I decided to study his case from another angle. I noticed that, as he fulfilled his obligations, he presented no difficulty to retain the urine, but when he sat down, he had to make a real effort to retain it.

Pulsatilla Nigricans patients get relief by moving. There are only few remedies that experiment relief by moving slowly, and Pulsatilla Nigricans and Ferum are the outstanding ones from this group.

Other symptoms are tearing, wounding pains relieved by movement and cold applications, and worsened by staying in warm rooms; dilatation of the veins in arms and hands; varicose veins in the limbs, similar to Acidum Fluoricum. Joint rheumatism and pain in limbs that have suffered a dislocation; sciatic pain which worsens at nights and ameliorates by walking slowly; tractions and tensions in the lower limbs muscles at nights when lying down; migrating tearing pains in the limbs.

Burning sensation in the veins and feet, it is necessary to get them out of the bed. The feet soles burn and hurt when walking. There is also unrest and contractions on the legs and feet; numb sensation in the leg on which the patient is leaning. Migratory pains in all the limbs.

Pulsatilla Nigricans Personality

- Has a good temper, is a shy and kind person
- Depends on other people's support
- Does not take decisions easily, insecure
- Makes friends easily
- Accepts other people's guidance
- Frequently weeps over anything and without reason
- Always are peaceful people
- Shy, sensitive children
- Is not direct for decision making
- Is a robust person
- Sometimes is blonde and thin
- He usually has light colored eyes
- Lack of confidence in himself
- Timid
- Weeps if someone speaks loudly, and feels better after crying without reason
- Changes from weeping to laughing
- Is an untidy person
- Easily becomes inhibited
- It is the most insecure personality among human beings
- He worries a lot, for everything and for everybody
- Fears the future and to carry out new activities
- Prefers to stay home
- It is a very skillful personality since it mentally changes from a topic to another
- Starts the day optimistic and it changes as the day goes by
- This personality faces great challenges with his weight, particularly if he belongs
- to the blood group "O"

7 Arsenicum Album

Anxiety, restlessness, depression, burning, foul or rotten smelling, cold pale body, sweaty and viscose skin. Excellent remedy, great aid for chronic diseases, accompanied by deep weakening'. Anxiety, restlessness, depression and fear.

Arsenicum Album affects several parts of the body: it seems to exaggerate or depress all its abilities, exciting and weakening all its functions.

The Arsenicum Album patient impresses medicine; only some symptoms prevail and they are important: anxiety, need to rest, depression, burning, foul smelling are typical. The body surface is pale and cold and it is covered by sweat. The patient has a hippocratic face in chronic conditions; it is accompanied by extreme weakness, such as anemia, malaria and malnutrition.

The anxiety in Arsenicum Album is accompanied by extreme fear, impulses, suicidal tendencies, sudden obsessions and whims. The patient is disappointed and shows different forms of excitement and delirium; when he is depressed, he is in an extraordinary mood. However, the patient is sometimes so sad that he does not want to live and wishes to die.

The Arsenicum Album patient moves constantly and changes postures frequently, if it is a child, he always wants to be with different people. While he is in bed, he is always changing positions and if possible, he wishes to leave his bed, as long as his weakness allows him to do so. There is great mental restlessness, worry about death, he cannot live straight and it is not the pain what leads him into this anguish, but his condition of deep depression. Among the main symptoms found in Arsenicum Album is a burning sensation in the brain which forces the patient to use cold water for showering and washing his face. The Arsenicum Album feels a burning sensation in the stomach, the vagina and the lungs; the patient feels he has a burning charcoal in these areas. Also, there is a burning feeling in the throat and in all the mucous membranes.

This patient also has a tendency for bleeding. He may bleed easily and any condition or symptom may cause such bleeding. He may vomit blood or suffer from throat hemorrhage or hematemesis. All bleedings occur due to inflammation of the mucous membranes. Likewise, hemorrhage is present in the bowels, kidneys, bladder and uterus; such discharge is black blood of putrid odor.

Usually the inflammations in Arsenicum Album are sudden and they are often malignant; such is the case of gangrenous inflammation of the lungs which provokes chills in the patient (Kent, Materia Médica).

The Arsenicum Album patient is always cold; he is always looking for a warm place since this makes him feel better sometimes. He covers up with clothes or blankets in order to keep warm. Most chronic disabled patients are unable to keep warm; they are usually pale with a wax like color. These patients also suffer from severe inflammatory conditions and hydropsy, thus suffering from periodic headaches, the more chronic their discomfort is the longer the cycle will last. Frequently, this condition worsens every seven days and in some patients with a deep, long—lasting and deeply rooted psora, though not serious, it may be present every two weeks (Kent, Materia Médica, Cuarta Edición, 1932).

In Arsenicum Album, the patient is very sensitive to odors and touch, thus making all senses exaggerate. Usually, this patient is bothered by confusion and lack of organization; he is extremely meticulous. There is diarrhea and flatulence. It is indicated for malaria and choleric conditions. There is an unbearable tenesmus, a terrible state of anxiety; the pain is so violent that the patient finds no other remedy than think about death.

The Arsenicum Album patient losses his voice (laryngitis), has a constant dry cough that can be overwhelming and torturing, which does not do any good. Relationship to asthma and dyspnea should be studied. The Arsenicum Album has cured cases of deeply rooted asthma (nervous type) appearing after midnight in cold, numb, pale patients. The whistling cough forces the patient to sit in bed pressing his thorax. There is an anxious restlessness and deep depression.

The heart symptoms are very difficult to handle if they are similar to the Arsenicum Album, since they appear in a condition of deep weakness. Strong heart beats occur with the_ slightest excitement or exercising. Extreme anxiety, anguish and weakness are also present. The patient is unable to climb stairs and walk, he can hardly move without having increased palpitations; all excitement causes a fast heart beating. Paroxysm due to the most severe heart conditions (incurable in many cases) and the similarity with the Arsenicum Album symptoms indicate the seriousness of the case: rheumatic angina pectoris, affecting the heart, hydropericarditis with increased irritability, small, frequent, shaking pulse and tremors all over the body.

Arsenicum Album Personality

- Restless, weak, and orderly
- They easily feel anguished and fatigued, they have a fragile appearance
- Very meticulous and perfectionist
- Order is of great importance for them
- Extremely hypoohondriac
- Fearful of being alone, fearful of death
- In senior citizens you will find that women always have their hair well done and make--up carefully applied. In men the same notion applies, he will be well groomed
- These personalities are usually very sensitive to cold; they get better with the normal heath of the environment
- They have a strong craving for cold things
- Both men and women show little expression
- They always have a high and mighty expression
- Almost always they are longilineal individuals, rarely obese
- When they sit down they are very well-mannered, they never lose poise
- These are the persons who never show their feelings in an expressive manner
- They are stoical people
- They are the most anxious and weak, sometimes malicious
- They have a tendency to be alone, away from civilization
- They improve with rest, they are easily depressed
- Violent; they get worse in a close room (claustrophobia)
- These people are always thirsty for large amounts of liquids, the colder the
- better

8 Lycopodium Clavatum

Strong religiousness: need to have an amulet to feel good.
Serious condition in cold weather. Prolapse of the uterus or the clitoris

Lycopodium Clavatum is a tri-miasmatic medicine (pscoric, psychotic, syphilitic). Its scope is broad and deep. It acts in soft tissues, blood vessels, bones, liver, heart, and joints where there could be necrosis, abscesses and ulcers. its prevalence is on the right side of the body; its symptoms migrate from left to right and from top to bottom (head—thorax). The patient loses weight in the upper half (neck in particular), while the lower extremities seem well nourished.

When there are symptoms of head and spine, there is sensitivity to heated environments. Head symptoms worsen by heat in the environment and in bed and also by exercise~induced flushing. The patient is sensitive to cold and shows a remarkable lack of vital heat; in general, the patient gets worse with cold temperature: with cold air, cold drinks and food. The pains are relieved by heat, except head and spine pains.

Generally, exercise aggravates the Lycopodium Clavatum patient: pants, gets upset and his dyspnea gets worse. It is impossible for him to climb and walk fast because his heart symptoms increase. Likewise, his dyspnea increases when he warms up due to exercise. The inflamed areas might be relieved by the application of heat, so does drinking tea or eating hot soup warms him up. Frequently, stomach symptoms are relieved by warm drinks or by warm substances arriving to the stomach. The agitation and deep depression are serious.

Regarding rheumatic pains and other ailments, the Lycopodium Clavatum patient is relieved by movement. He is extremely restless, constantly tossing and turning, and when there is inflammation with pain and suffering, his bed is a refuge and movement relieves, that is why he tosses and turns all night. He turns and makes himself comfortable in a new place thinking he will be able to sleep but his unease continues all night.

When the patient has headache symptoms, he needs cold air; he needs to stay in a cool place. Even if a headache gets worse with movement, enough to flush the patient, it does not get worse by movement itself. A headache gets worse when lying down and with a room's hot temperature. it improves with cold air and movement, just until the patient has moved and exercise enough to get warmed up then the headache worsens.

The Lycopodium Clavatum patient is flatulent and distended like a drum, so much that sometimes he has breathing difficulties. His diaphragm, pushing upward, invades the space of the lungs and the heart so that, he suffers palpitations, fainting and dyspnea. It is not a rare occurrence to hear a Lycopodium Clavatum patient say: "Everything I eat turns into gas". After eating no more than a mouthful he becomes flatulent and so distended he is unable to eat any more. The patient reports that a single mouthful has filled him up to his throat. He will feel as nervous as to be unable to stand any noise. The rustle of a paper, the sound of bells, or the noise of a slamming door will cause fainting spells as in Antimonium Crudum, Borax and Natrum Muriatioum. These general conditions are present in all the ailments, acute and chronic. All his senses are excited, everything upsets him, and any insignificance will bother him making him feel bad.

The skin ulcerates; there are painful, sloughing ulcers and abscesses under the skin, as well cell disorder. The chronic ulcerations are indolent and they are paired with false granulation. They hurt, burn, sting and itch and are often relieved by applying cold compresses but worsen with hot dressings.

In a general sense, it is true that heat and warm dressings relieve the Lycopodium Clavatum patient. Warm compresses relieve knee pain, suppurating condition, and gout disorders. In a very warm bed or in a heated room hives come out either in nodules or in long and irregular stripes, with violent itching. The Lycopodium Clavatum has eruptions upon the skin that itch violently. The patient also has vesicles and scaly eruptions moist and dry or furfuraceous eruptions, eruptions around the lips, behind the ears, under the wings of the nose and upon the genitals; fissured eruptions, bleeding fissures like salt rheum upon the hands.

The skin becomes thick and indurate. The sites of old boils and pustules become indurate and form nodules that remain a long time. The skin looks unhealthy, and it will slough easily. Wounds will not heal, surface wounds suppurate as if they had contained splinters, and this suppuration burrows along under the skin.

The Lycopodium Clavatum state when deciphered shows feebleness throughout: arteries and veins are too relaxed, their tone and circulation poor. There is numbness in certain spots. Emaciation of some members, there is no numbness of the fingers and toes. There is staggering and inability, clumsiness and awkwardness as well as trembling of the limbs.

The Lycopodium Clavatum has a religious mania, which has a mild and simple beginning, a matter of melancholy. This religious melancholy grows greater and greater until he sits and broods. He has aversion to company however, he dreads solitude. "Dread of men and dread of solitude; irritability and melancholy." This dread of men is not always a state of dread in women, it is a certain dread of people, that when it is fully expressed in a Lycopodium Clavatum patient you will see that she dreads the presence of strangers, or the arriving of friends or visitors, she does not want to make any kind of exertion, yet at times, when forced to do so she is relieved. Taciturnity, desires to be alone.

Let us follow that a little further. The taciturnity is because the patient does not want to talk. She wants to keep silent, but as I have already said, she feels very glad there is somebody else in the house and that she is no alone. She is perfectly willing to remain in a little room by herself, so that she is practically alone, yet not in solitude. if there were two adjacent rooms in the house you would find the Lycopodium Clavatum patient staying in one of them but very pleased to know there is someone else in the other.

The Lycopodium patient often cries when receiving a friend of meeting an
acquaintance. On the event of receiving a gift she feels a strange sadness with weeping.

Children are lean, emaciated and suffer prolonged headaches. Every time
they are exposed to cold they have headaches, prolonged, throbbing congestion from day to day and from month to month. They become more emaciated, especially

about the face and neck. This ailment is also present when narrow chested boys have a dry, annoying cough, without expectoration, whose face and neck emaciates. This remedy is particularly suitable in those thin girls with a dry cough and prolonged headache. In children who lose weight after pneumonia or bronchitis, and emaciate about the face and the neck, catch colds on the slightest provocation and suffer headaches from being heated; children who also suffer nightly headaches, and a certain state of congestion that more or less affects the mind and in which they wake up in confusion. The child screams out in sleep, awakes frightened, looks wild, and does not recognize his parents or relatives until after a few moments when he seems to be able to recover his senses and realizes where he is and then goes back to bed and falls asleep again. After a little while, he wakes up frightened again, looks strange and confused. This behavior repeats again.

Lycopodium Clavatum suffers from thick, yellow discharge from the nose. The nose is filled with yellow, green crusts, which are blown out of the nose or hawked out of the throat in the morning. Now then, when the patient takes cold, the tick discharge ceases significantly, he starts to sneeze and has a watery discharge, then follows a headache.

Lycopodium Clavatum has become an important remedy for the ears because that very same emaciating child, with contorted countenance and dry cough, has had attacks of scarlet fever and a thick, yellow, offensive discharge from the ears, with loss of hearing. In the case of scarlet fever where the suitable remedy has been given, since those troubles do not necessarily belong to scarlet fever, they are no a part of it. They are dependent on the constitutional state of the child. Lycopodium Clavatum has also the most painful eruptions of the ears, otitis media, and abscesses in the ear, associated with eczema on and behind the ears.

The next important noticeable feature in the Lycopodium Clavatum symptoms is the throat. It was mentioned when going over the general state pointing out that the main feature of the Lycopodium Clavatum in regard to direction is that its symptoms seem to spread from right to left. We mentioned that the right foot is cold and the left is warm. The right knee is the affected one and the pains are migratory, going from right to left. Most of the pains of the remedy seem to travel this way or affect the right side more than the left. This is also true, of sore throats: a quinsy affecting the right side when its course has about ended will have caused the left tonsil to become inflamed and tosuppurate if the appropriate remedy has not been administered. The common sore throat will start on the right side, the next day both sides will be affected, when the inflammation has extended to the left side.

The Lycopodium Clavatum has a wide range of pains in the larynx and maxillary.

The gastric and abdominal symptoms are intermingled. There is a particular sense of satiety, and a total lack of appetite. The patient feels so full that he cannot eat. This sense of satiety may not appear until he has eaten something. He sits at the table feeling hungry, after eating, he is distended with flatus, and although he gets momentary relief from belching, he remains distended. There is nausea and vomiting of bile, coffee ground vomit, and black inky vomit. Apparently malignant cases treated with Lycopodium Clavatum have their life prolonged, instead of culminating in a few months the patient may last for years. The right hypochondrium is swollen as in liver troubles.

There is pain in the liver,_recurrent bilious attacks with vomiting of bile. He suffers from colic due to gall stones. Once Lycopodium Clavatum is administered the attacks will be less frequent, the bilious secretion will become normal and the gall stones will have a spongy appearance as though they were being dissolved with a strong urge to defecate. There are sharp pains in the liver region, an urging to defecate with no results or insufficient and slow results and with ball—like stool. Mucous or blood. Prolapsed intestine (cloaca) with itching and burning sensation. Urine suppression with pain and sharp burning in the urethra. There is precocious, insufficient or suppressed menstruation. Discharge of mucous or yellowish or greenish red secretion, or fetid pus from the clitoris, with itching, excoriation and eczema.

Pain decreases with strenuous exercise and increases when resting in the afternoon and at night, constipation pain in the lower abdomen, a gestational the menstruation at a critical age; irregularities in venous flow. There is yellow, gray, pain as a consequence of suppressing sweat in feet, of suppression of or liver–colored spotting of the skin, especially on the face, chest, or stomach region. This is especially present in irritable—tempered and easily excited people who are prone to sadness, anguishing concerns and health issues. There is a misanthropic irritability and bad temper, together with a weak memory.

The Lycopodium Clavatum Personality

- Insecure, proud, possessive and jealous
- Alternate between self-assurance and insecurity
- Cry, or make faces at the slightest provocation
- Always want to be the first in everything
- Listen to music, feel nostalgia and might end up crying
- Eternally in love, they fall in love with everything
- If they eat out, they eat always at the same place until bored or fed up
- If they buy a piece of clothing and they like it, they buy more
- They are extravagant in taste as they are in their vanity
- If they arrive to a party or reunion they want to stand out and shine and they know how to do it
- Extremely nervous, sometimes they lack confidence in themselves
- On occasion, they are the most self-assured people in the world
- When they get angry, they get to the point where they are unable to manage their anger
- They regret what they have done, immediately
- Jealous, so much that they follow their love one
- They have an exaggerated need for affection
- As a father or a mother they tend to be possessive and jealous
- Exaggerate; they exaggerate any accomplishment at a thousand percent
- Almost always they suffer from hangnails (cuticles detach from the fingernails)
- Always need to be accompanied by someone
- Do not accept the slightest contradiction
- Sexually, they are more solicitous, they can be promiscuous and impotent. They can be concerned for their partner or do without it. In privacy they are very jealous and pathologically shy They always live and remember their past (they live in it)

- They are real fighters
- Always looking for a way to prosper
- They are afraid of the future and of failure
- They have a religious attitude
- Sometimes they are malicious
- Many times, they get what they aim at, convincing by means of words or actions
- When they speak they omit _syllab|es or words
- They have a bad memory, especially short term memory
- Extremely resentful, never forget anything that hurts or has hurt them
- They are not direct on theirjudgments
- If they are eating, and for example, a poor and needy person is beside them, they will share their food or clothes

Appendix I

Dr. Christian Friedrich Samuel Hahnemann
Chronology of the most important events in his
professional career.

1755. Born in Meissen (Saxony), on April 10.

1767 to1775. Already renowned in his school for his fast progress in Natural Sciences, his teachers give him a free entry to all the school courses, considering his parents were poor.

1779. Completes his doctorate on August 10, publicly presenting his thesis: Conspectus affectum spasmodicorum cerfilogicus et therapeuticus, at the University of Earlangen. A

1787. Hahnemann was appointed Chief Doctor in the Military Hospital.

1789. Hahnemann absolutely abandoned the practice of allopathic medicine, devoting himself to chemistry studies.

1790. He publishes his exposition on the way to prepare soluble mercury, and begins his homeopathic studies.

1794. In Komlgsluther he obtains amazing cures with his system never before seen by the allopathic system. Pharmacist started to oppose as a result he gained the attention of the medical and profane world and had to move to Albona. Publishes his findings on the properties of Belladonna.

1796. Publishes his essay on the new way to approach the knowledge of medicinal properties.

1800. In a Scarlet fever epidemic in Germany he obtains great success with belladonna.

1801. Publishes his healing and preservative method for scarlet fever and a pamphlet on the medical confraternity at the beginning of the new century.

1803. Publishes an opuscule on coffee and its effect.

1804. Publishes two volumes in Leipzig titled Fragmenta de viribus medicamentorum positivis sive in sano corpore humana observatis.

1805. Publishes in Berlin another book titled The Medicine Experience,

developed in his Organon.

1808. Publishes in Torgan his treatise "On the value of Speculative System of Medicine" '

1810. Publishes the first edition of his book Organon of the Rational An' of Healing". '

1811. Publishes in Leipzig his six volumes of The doctrine of Pure Pharmacology

1813. Gives homeopathy oral lessons in Leipzig, and sustains publicly his thesis Disertatio hitorico-medica de Heleborismo-reterum, making there pure experiences on homeopathy turning remedies into substances and tinctures.

1814. Publishes his new method to fight the prevailing typhus fever.

1816. Publishes, in Leipzig his Memories on Syphilis.

1820. Hahnemann is summoned to court for having administered homeopathic medicine. His brilliant defense is published in the General Homeopathic Gazette.

1821. Hahnemann and other homeopaths are authorized to administer their remedies in Leipzig.

1822. Hahnermann accepts the position of private doctor for the Duke of Anhalt Goethen.

1823. Publishes his Instruction for those searching for the truth, and The best way to make the homeopathic method disappear.

1828–1830 In Dresden he publishes his "Chronic Diseases, their Peculiar Nature and Homoeopathic Treatment". In that period he started his medical dynamism.

1829. Publishes a writing entitled The chronic diseases, their peculiar nature and homeopathic treatment, in that year all the homeopaths of different countries met in Dresden for the first time to celebrate the anniversary of Hahnemann's doctorate.

1830. Hahnemann cures, successfully, the cholera sufferers.

1835. On June 25 he moves to Paris and settles there definetily.

1843. Hahnemann dies in Paris, on July 2.

1851. A statue was build in Leipzig

Apendix II

Invocation

Almighty God, inspire me with love for my art and for Thy creatures. Do not allow thirst for profit, ambition for renown and admiration, to interfere with my profession. Preserve the strength of my body and of my soul that they ever be ready to cheerfully help and support rich and poor, good and bad, enemy as well as friend. '

In the sufferer let me see only the human being. Illumine my mind that it recognize what presents itself and that it may comprehend what is absent or hidden. Let it not fail to see what is visible, but do not permit it to arrogate to itself the power to see what cannot be seen, for delicate and indefinite are the bounds of the great art of caring for the lives and health of Thy creatures.

Grant that my patients have confidence in me and my art and follow my directions and my counsel.

Remove from their midst all charlatans and the whole host of officious relatives and know-all nurses, cruel people who arrogantly frustrate the wisest purposes of our art and often lead Thy creatures to their death.

Grant me God Almighty, indulgence and patience with the obstinate and rude patients.

Let me be contented in everything except in the great science of my profession. For art is great, but the mind of man is ever expanding. Never allow the thought to arise in me that I have attained to sufficient knowledge, but vouchsafe to me the strength, the leisure and the ambition ever to extend my knowledge so that it may benefit those who suffer.

Amen!

Moses Ben Maimonides, The Spaniard

www.ingramcontent.com/pod-product-compliance
Lightning Source LLC
Chambersburg PA
CBHW070917180526
45168CB00005B/2046